Happy Together
a sperm donation story

Written by Julie Marie
Illustrated by Ashley Lucas

This book is dedicated to JLN,

as promised many years ago.

Copyright © 2019 Julie Marie

All rights reserved. No part of this publication may be reproduced, stored in a retrieval system, or transmitted, in any form or by any means, electronic, mechanical, photocopying, recording or otherwise without the prior written permission from the copyright owner.

ISBN-13: 978-1-7333572-1-0

ISBN-10: 1-7333572-1-1

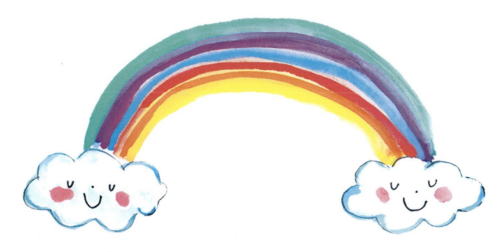

Happy Together

a sperm donation story

Written by Julie Marie

Illustrated by Ashley Lucas

Years ago, the sun was shining bright one day
The sky was blue above,

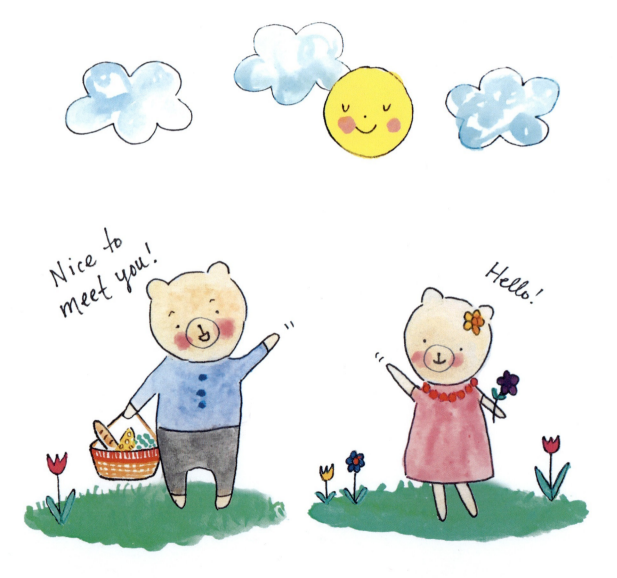

That's when Mommy and Daddy met each other
And then we fell in love.

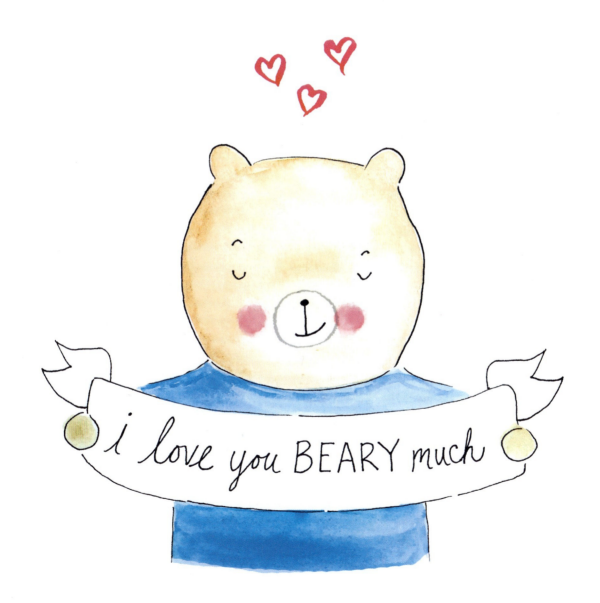

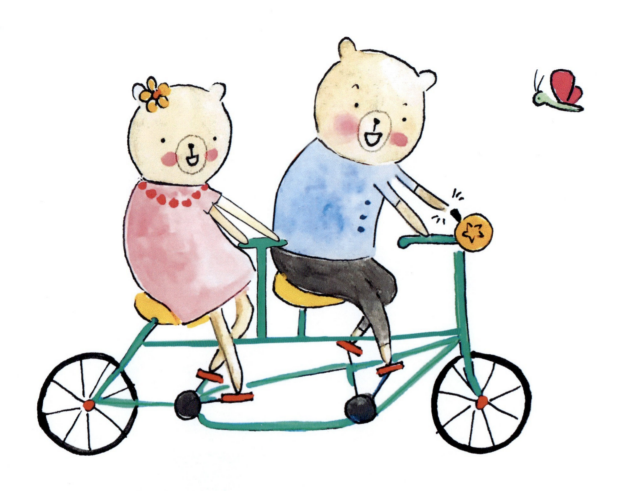

We went on many adventures
Laughing, smiling and having fun,

Mommy and Daddy married
Our life together had just begun.

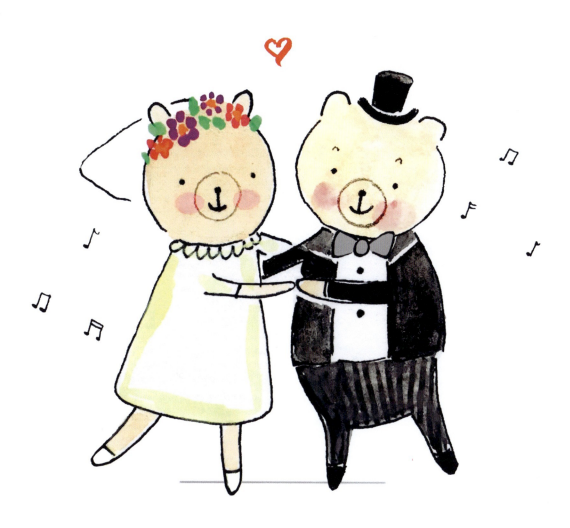

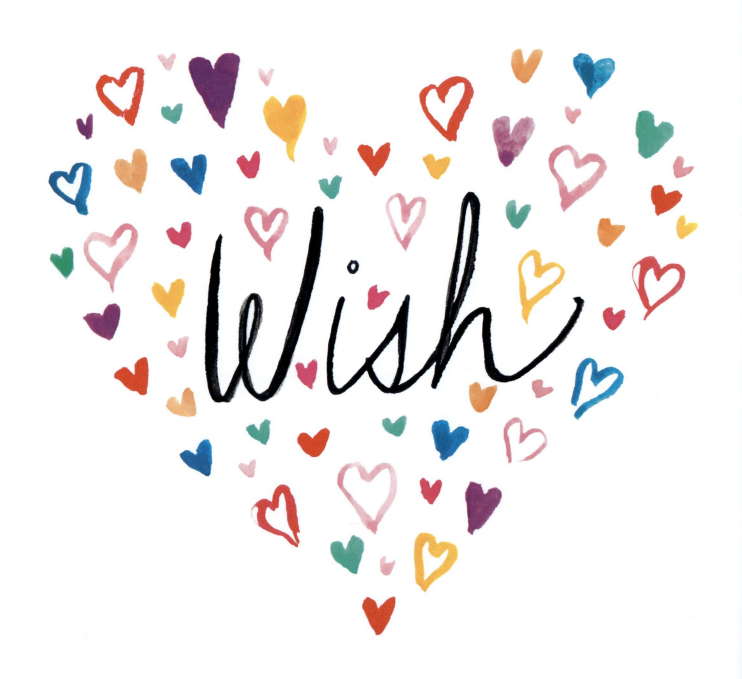

Deep within our hearts
We had a special wish
More than anything, we wanted to have a baby
To love, hug and kiss!

For some Mommies and Daddies
It's easy to have a baby
And for some Mommies and Daddies
It takes a lot.
For your Mommy and Daddy
Our journey to have you
Would take longer than we thought...

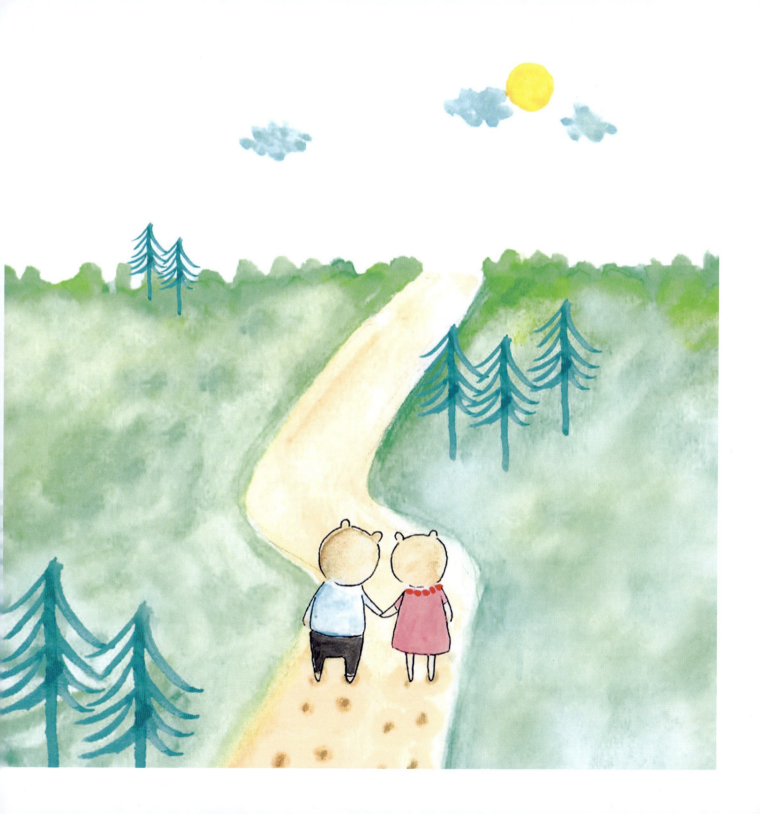

Time passed and there was no baby
We needed to try something new
We went to a doctor for help
And never gave up on our dream of having you.

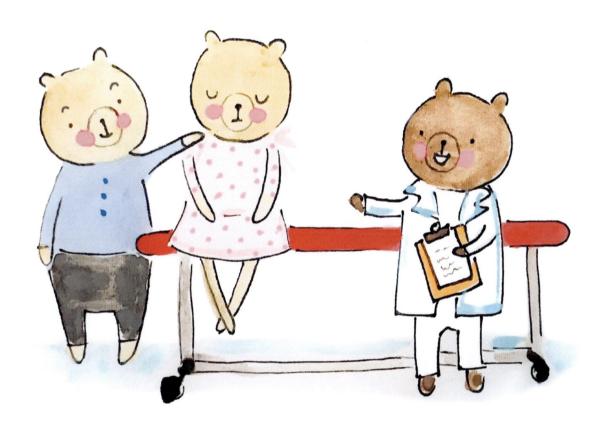

Mommy and Daddy went to the doctor many times
Mommy took lots of medicine
As the seasons passed by

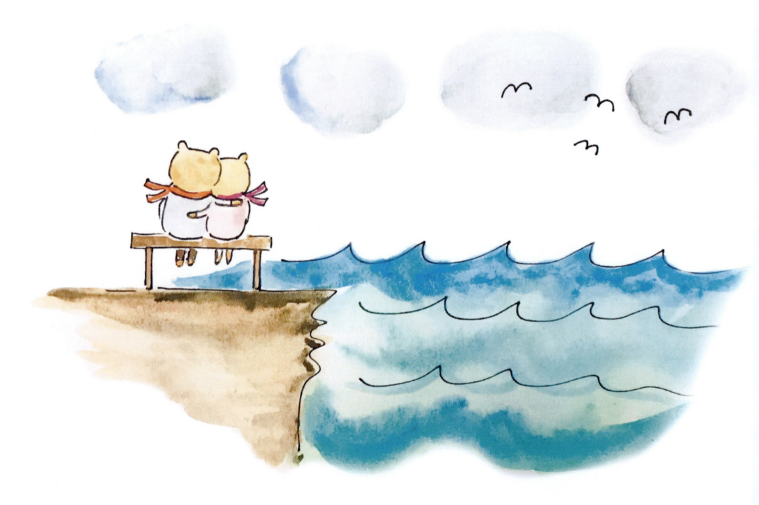

The medicine didn't work and we were so sad...

But the doctor knew of something else we could try!

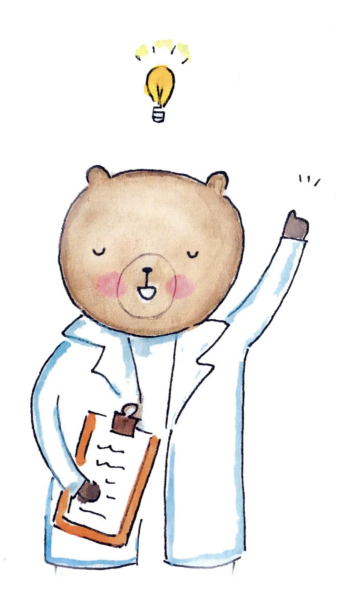

To make a baby
It takes an egg from Mommy
And a seed from Daddy
But Daddy's seeds weren't working
And couldn't make a baby.
We needed a new plan,

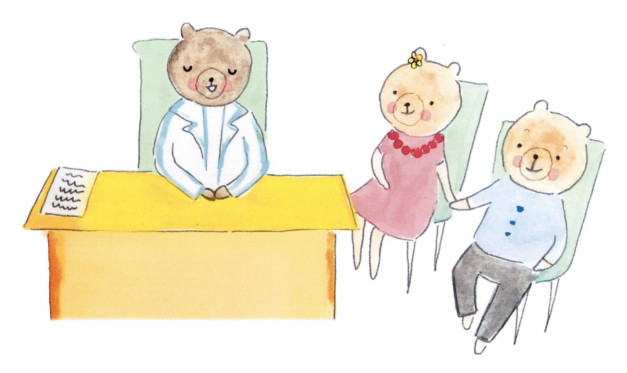

It was then we asked for the help of a very special man.

The special man is called a donor,
and he gave the very important gift of a seed

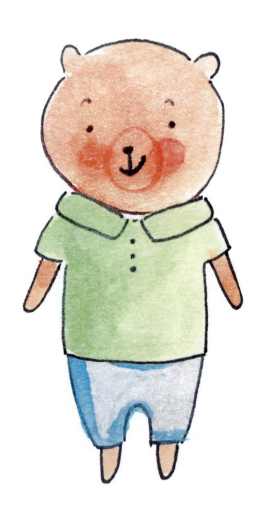

The doctor helped Mommy's egg
combine with the donor's seed

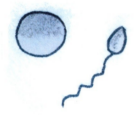

And it turned out to be exactly what
we would need!

Once again, the sun was shining bright one day
The sky was blue above
That's when Mommy and Daddy received the best news
Mommy was pregnant with you
And our hearts were full of love!

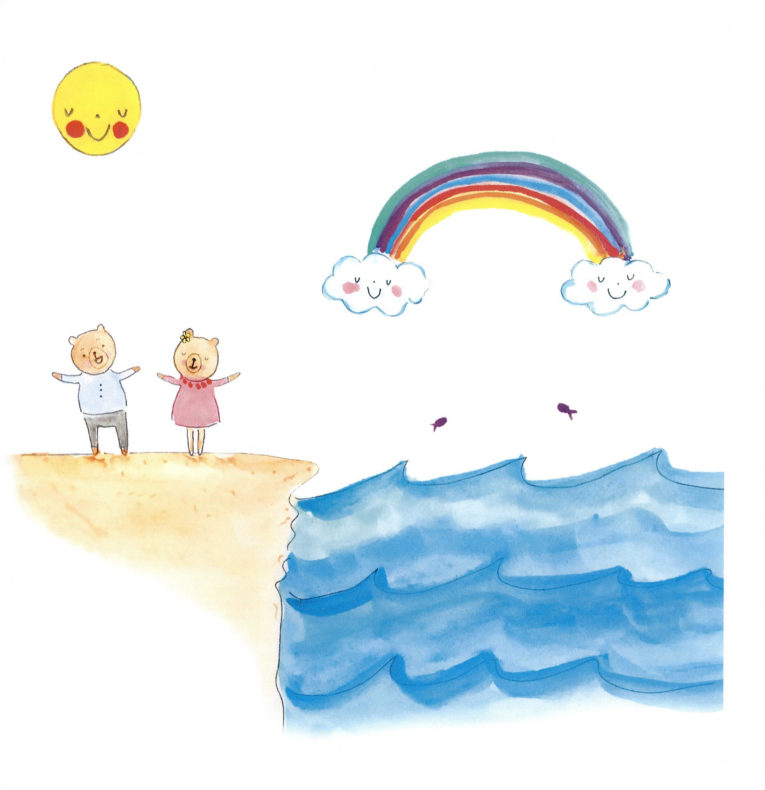

As the months passed by
Bigger and bigger Mommy's tummy grew,

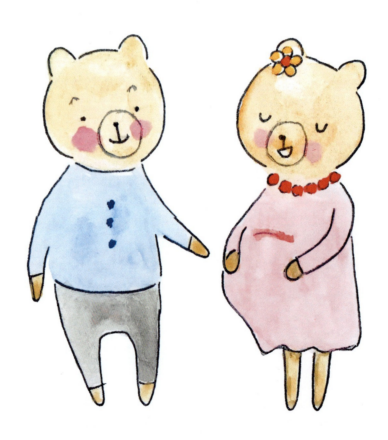

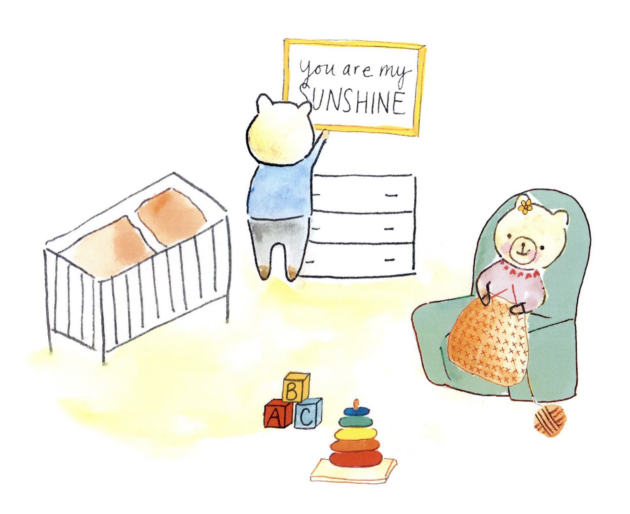

We cheerfully prepared for your arrival
We were so excited to meet you!

The day you were born
Our dream of having a child came true,

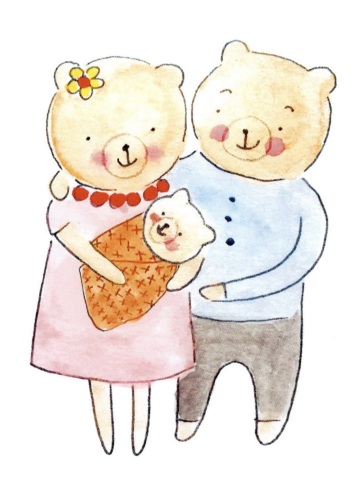

Mommy and Daddy were beyond grateful
To finally be able to love, hug and kiss you!

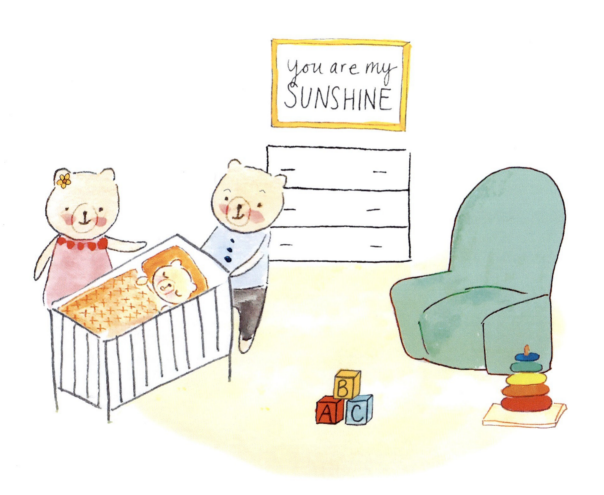

Happy together, we are a family
Mommy and Daddy's love for you is beyond measure,

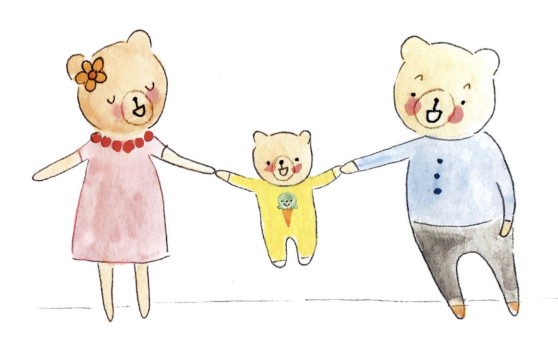

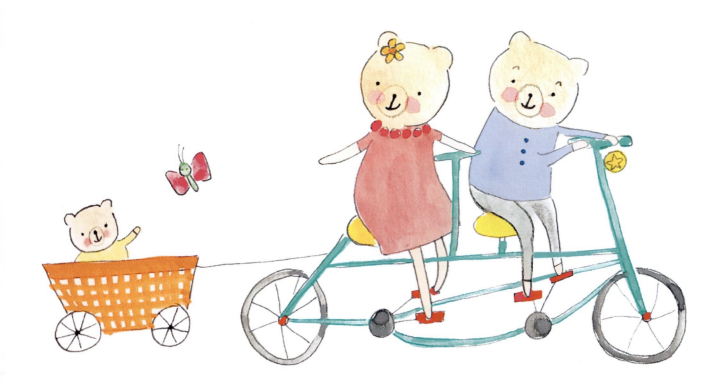

We laugh, smile and have fun
Making memories we will always treasure!

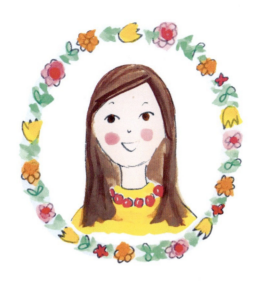

JULIE MARIE

I am an infertility advocate
and mother through IVF.

It is my hope that Happy Together
will provide a heartwarming,
family building story for parents
to read with their child
sharing just how much they were
wished for and loved.